KETO

MW01491065

MEAL PREP

COOKBOOK

The Ultimate Weight Loss Guide

For Beginners With The Best

And Easy Recipes

Written by: Luisa Grant

Copyright © 2018

All rights reserved.

The information contained in **"Keto Meal Prep Cookbook,"** and its components, is meant to serve as a comprehensive collection of strategies that the author of this Book has done research about. Summaries, strategies, tips and tricks are only recommendations by the author, and reading this Book will not guarantee that one's results will exactly mirror the author's results.

The author of this book has made all reasonable efforts to provide current and accurate information for the readers of this Book. The author and its associates will not be held liable for any unintentional errors or omissions that may be found.

The material in the book may include information by third parties. Third party materials comprise of opinions expressed by their owners. As such, the author of this Book does not assume responsibility or liability for any third party material or opinions.

The publication of third party material does not constitute the author's guarantee of any information, products, services, or opinions contained within third party material. Use of third party material does not guarantee that your results will mirror our results. Publication of such third party material is simply a recommendation and expression of the author's own opinion of that material.

Whether because of the progression of the Internet, or the unforeseen changes in company policy and editorial submission guidelines, what is stated as fact at the time of this writing may become outdated or inapplicable later.

This book is copyright ©2018 by **Luisa Grant** with all rights reserved. It is illegal to redistribute, copy, or create derivative works from this Ebook whole or in parts. No parts of this report may be reproduced or retransmitted in any forms whatsoever without the written expressed and signed permission from the author.

TABLE OF CONTENTS

Introduction

The list of ketogenic diet benefits is a long, happy one. Here's what to **expect the first month** after switching to a ketogenic diet plan.

As a side note, I would encourage you to get a full blood lipid panel done before starting the plan, so that you can compare the results of your blood work before and afterwards.

- Reduction in blood triglycerides: carbohydrate consumption is closely tied to triglyceride levels, and one of most well known ketogenic diet benefits. The less carbohydrate you eat, the lower your triglycerides readings will go. The ratio of triglycerides to HDL (expressed Triglyceride/HDL) is the best predictor of heart attack risk and is one of blood test results to which you should really pay attention. The closer this ratio is to 1:1, the healthier you are. See this paper.
- Reduction of total cholesterol: Cholesterol is made from excess glucose in the diet. As you eat less sugar creating foods, you do less damage to your arterial system and inflammation drops. Your cholesterol will drop as your body has less glucose from which to make it, and less need for repairing the damages of inflammatory chemicals.
- Increase in HDL Cholesterol (the more saturated fat you eat, the higher it will go.) This is actually a good thing, because it improves the ratio of HDL/LDL. Higher HDL levels (above 39 mg/dL) indicate a healthier heart.
- Reduction in fasting blood sugar and fasting insulin levels: As you eat less carb, there is less sugar driving up blood sugar and insulin levels.
- Freedom from hypoglycemia, food fixations and sugar cravings. This is by far the best benefit in my opinion. Having control over your eating habits is so empowering.
- Lack of hunger: Ketone bodies dampen the appetite, and fat is very satisfying. You'll notice at times, you may forget to eat. You may find this is the most amazing part, especially if you struggle with food addiction issues.
- Lower blood pressure: Low carb diets are very effective at reducing blood pressure. If you are taking any blood pressure medications, be aware that you might start feeling dizzy from too much medication while on a ketogenic diet plan. You may be able to reduce your BP meds (talk to your doctor first).
- Reduction in blood levels of C Reactive Protein (CRP) and HbA1c proteins: These are both markers of inflammation and heart disease risk.

- More energy. You'll be amazed at how much energy you have. Any chronic fatigue symptoms should get better. If you are taking a statin (a cholesterol lowering drug) see my statin side effects page. Statins compromise cellular mitochondria which results in fatigue and muscle pain.
- Clearer thinking. The "fogginess" that accompanies a high carb diet will disappear. My theory on this is that the brain is over 60% fat by weight, and the more fat you eat, the better it can maintain itself and work to its full capacity. Others more scientifically inclined might talk about essential fatty acids and neurotransmitter function.
- Heartburn relief: if you suffer from GERD or other heartburn issues, the symptoms should lessen or disappear. Heartburn, I believe, is a direct result of eating grain based foods, sugar and for some people, nightshade vegetables such as tomatoes. I also believe it is tied to problems with sleep apnea, as described above in the sleep section.
- Changes in your sleep patterns and an improvement in sleep apnea symptoms. I believe that sleep apnea is tied to grain consumption, the heartburn it causes, and reactive hypoglycemia from a high carb diet. I used to have apnea, but once I cut grains out of my diet and permanently reduced my carb intake, I no longer have it, just as I no longer get heartburn or hypoglycemia. Another sleep benefit of eating less carbs is that those urges to take a late afternoon nap will go away. Not falling asleep at your desk every afternoon is one of the best ketogenic diet benefits.
- Weight loss: sticking to a ketogenic diet plan can be very effective for normalizing your weight. However, if you have very high fasting insulin (and high insulin resistance) you may need to add a high intensity exercise program like Doug McGuff's Body by Science: A Research Based Program to Get the Results You Want in 12 Minutes a Week. High intensity training has the effect of increasing the insulin sensitivity of your muscles, thereby decreasing your fasting insulin and help you lose weight. While one of the most common ketogenic diet benefits is weight loss, it may not be as easy as it has been advertised for some. Most people who are very heavy have very broken metabolisms. However, they are also the people who are most likely to experience many of ketogenic diet benefits. I am one of those people. My story on how I got healthy, fixed my metabolism and lost weight will give you an idea of what might be involved.
- Decrease in stiffness and joint pain. This is one of the best side effects of following a ketogenic diet plan. The diet eliminates grain based foods from your diet, and they,

in my opinion are the biggest cause of chronic illness and pain, especially muscle stiffness and joint pain. As I often say, no grain, no pain.

- Gum disease and tooth decay: sugar changes the pH of your mouth and contributes to tooth decay. Three months into a ketogenic diet, any gum disease you might have will decrease or disappear.
- Digestion and gut health get better. You will see a decrease in stomach pain, bloating, gas etc.. These are all associated with grain and sugar consumption.
- Mood stabilization. Ketone bodies have been shown to be beneficial in stabilizing neurotransmitters such as serotonin and dopamine which result in better mood control.
- As you can see from the list above, the temporary unpleasant effects of switching to a ketogenic diet are totally worth it when you experience the many ketogenic diet benefits.
- If you have any lingering concerns, please remember that the latest scientific studies (here's a list) have shown that following a ketogenic diet plan is not detrimental to human health, if it is eaten while also minimizing carbohydrate intake. This is the key to experiencing the long list of ketogenic diet benefits: eat a diet low in carbs, high in natural fats, and moderate in protein intake.
- It's only when you combine lots of fat and lots of carbohydrates in your diet that you get into trouble. The sugar from the carbohydrates drives up your insulin levels, and those high insulin levels cause any fat you eat to be stored immediately. This causes the weight gain associated with insulin resistance and starts the health problems that should be associated with a high carb diet.

Saves money

Eating homemade foods is usually much cheaper than eating at a restaurant or buying processed foods from the market.

"When we eat at a restaurant, we pay for not only the food, but also the costs of running that business. The lights, the water, the building, and the staff — in addition to the meal we are eating. The same goes for the pre-made or frozen meals at grocery stores."

Here are some additional ways Ben suggests to save money:

- Plan several days of meals. We'll be less likely be tempted to eat something else if we have a plan or something already made.
- Make a grocery list and stick to it to avoid buying extra food.
- Save leftovers in the refrigerator or freezer. Once you get a stock of leftovers stored, you can reheat them at a later date when you don't have time to cook.

Saves time

It might seem like grabbing something to eat at the local supermarket or driving to get take-out at the closest restaurant might be a quick solution when you're in a hurry. In reality, many times it can be much faster to cook something at home, especially when you plan ahead. There are so many meals that can be made in less than 30 minutes. And if you choose a more complex recipe, you can always cook in bulk and eat the surplus later in the week or freeze it.

Healthier ingredients

Many commercially prepared foods are high in fat, salt, and sugar. When we prepare our own food, we know exactly which ingredients and how much of each are going into our food.

"When we cook at home, we are in control. McDonald's fries have 19 ingredients. We can make them at home with far less — and they will taste just as good. A favorite at my house is potatoes cut into wedges, olive oil, salt, pepper, and cayenne pepper. Put these in a Ziploc bag to mix together. Then place in the oven on a pan for about 30 minutes at 400 F. It's only five ingredients, and tastes fabulous."

Avoid food allergies and sensitivities

Preparing your food at home can be especially beneficial if you or a family member has a food allergy. Because you are in control in your own kitchen, you can reduce the risk of an allergic reaction.

Portion control

Many restaurants and fast food joints offer portions that are much larger than necessary. And the problem is, when food is in front of you, chances are you'll eat it. When you dine in, you can regulate the amount of food served for dinner, eliminating unnecessary temptation.

Brings family together

Eating at home gives the entire family time to talk about their day.

"Studies show that when we eat together, our kids and family are much healthier. Eating together is linked to less obesity, kids doing better in school, and less substance abuse within the family."

Involving your children in food preparation (maybe by asking them to read the recipe out loud or mix ingredients) is not only a fun thing to do, but also a great way to teach them healthy eating habits.

How to Pack Your Meal

1. Stock up on containers.

There is no way around this — in order to pack a week's worth of lunches, you are going to need a week's worth of containers. Buying a set or two of matching lunch boxes will make stacking and stashing packed lunches in the fridge easier, but you can also utilize mismatched pieces if needed. Small containers for salad dressings or dips will be helpful too.

2. Embrace repetition.

To save time (and your sanity), repeat a few of the same lunch components throughout the week. Monday's salad Avocado with breast can also be packed as a side for Thursday's turkey wrap.

3. Pack some things frozen.

Yogurt freezes well and, whether you freezer yogurt squeeze-tubes or package your own yogurt, freezing it will keep the yogurt from sloshing about in the lunch box. Apple sauce transports better this way too. Corn, peas, and cooked edamame can all go into lunch boxes frozen and they will thaw in the fridge, which keeps them fresher longer.

4. Know what will last.

Understanding what recipes are worthy of packing for a week's worth of lunches takes some trial and error. While that doesn't mean certain foods are unable to be packed ahead, it does require some strategic planning. For example, sliced strawberries will be mushy by midweek, so they should go into Monday or Tuesday's box.

5. Leave a few things unpacked.

While the goal for packing a week's worth of lunches is to eliminate the daily chore of packing lunches, it is OK to leave a few packing details for the day of. Browned avocados aren't appetizing to most eaters, so while you can pack up the black bean salad, quesadilla, and watermelon for Tuesday's lunch on Sunday afternoon, you should hold off on slicing and packing the avocado until Tuesday morning. I like to give apples the same treatment.

6. Pack while you cook.

Let me be straight with you: Packing a week's worth of lunches is going to make a mess of your kitchen, so better to pair it with a meal you can enjoy afterwards and only do cleanup once. Another bonus? You'll already have the oven on for roasting vegetables or toasting frozen waffles.

7. Take shortcuts.

Here is your permission to rely on ready-made meal components, in case you needed it. Find frozen waffles you love and use them to make sandwiches, or serve breakfast for lunch; pack your favorite store-bought dressing; or use pre-made pizza dough to make pizza pinwheels.

8. Don't overfill lunch boxes.

Squishing food into too tight a space is a surefire shortcut to spoilage. Salad greens packed too densely can't breath and will start to wilt; stacked and squished sandwiches will get soggy. This is where a bento-style container with compartments comes in hand — each component of lunch can be packed in its own space without squishing against each other.

9. Pack wet things separately.

Chicken salad sandwiches - packing chicken salad on bread just means soggy sandwiches by midweek. Instead pack the chicken salad and the bread in separate compartments. Same goes for salad dressings. Packing mayo for sandwiches on the side as well as sauces for cold noodles will ensure tasty lunches from Monday through Friday.

DAY 1

Breakfast: Casserole with Sausage

Prep + Cooking time: 15 minutes

Servings: 4

Ingredients:

- 1 pound Italian Sausage
- 4 Egg whites
- 2 Eggs
- 2/3 cup of Reduced sodium veggie broth
- 2/3 cup of cheese, jam-packed (2.5 oz)
- 1/4 cup of Pesto sauce of preference
- 1/4 cup of Roasted red pepper, sliced
- 1/4 tablespoon of sea salt
- Pinch of chili
- 4 tablespoon of Pine nut products, minced
- Fresh basil

Directions:

1. Preheat oven to 400 degrees.
2. Heat a medium skillet on medium temperature and prepare the sausage, frequently stirring, until fantastic brown.
3. Once grilled, drain off extra fat and pass on it into the lower part of the skillet.
4. Pour the sausage.
5. Bake before eggs puffs up.

6. Garnish with the pine nut products and basil and serve!

Lunch: Blt Chicken Breast Salad Stuffed Avocados

Prep + Cooking time: 15 minutes

Servings: 6

Ingredients:

- 12 pieces of turkey bacon (3 reds)
- 1 1/2 mugs shredded rotisserie fowl (2 reds)
- 2 Roma tomato (1 green)
- 1 1/2 mugs cottage cheese
- 1 cup finely sliced romaine lettuce (1 green)
- 3 avocados

Directions:

1. Preheat your oven to 400 degrees.
2. Bake 12 pieces of turkey bacon for ten minutes, turn, bake for another 5 minutes, and place the bacon out over several layers of paper towels to cool.
3. Cut your tomato vegetables, scoop out all the pulp and seed products with your fingertips, and dice into small chunks.
4. Chop the romaine into small pieces.
5. In a sizable bowl, incorporate the cottage mozzarella cheese, chicken, romaine, tomato vegetables, crumbled turkey bacon, and mix together.
6. Season to style with sodium and pepper.
7. Serve.

Dinner: Bangin' Coconut-Lime Skirt Steak

Prep + Cooking time: 30 minutes

Servings: 2

Ingredients:

- 1/2 glass coconut oil, melted
- zest of 1 lime
- 2 tablespoon of newly squeezed lime drink in one lime
- 1 tablespoon of minced garlic
- 1 teaspoon of grated fresh ginger
- 1 teaspoon of red pepper flakes
- 3/4 teaspoon of sea salt
- 2lb grass given skirt steak

Directions:

1. In a sizable bowl, Mix the coconut oil, lime and zest, garlic clove, ginger, red pepper flakes and sodium.
2. Add the steak toss.
3. Let meats marinate for approximately 20 minutes at room temperatures.
4. Pour steak into a huge skillet place over medium-high warmth.
5. Slice and Serve!

DAY 2

Breakfast: Keto Waffles

Prep + Cooking time: 10 minutes

Servings: 3

Ingredients:

- 3 eggs - medium separated
- 2.4 tablespoon of coconut flour
- 2.4 tablespoon of granulated sweetener
- 0.6 tablespoon of cooking powder
- 1.2 tablespoon of vanilla
- 1.8 tablespoon of full fats dairy or cream
- 75g of melted butter

Directions:

1. First bowl: Whisk the egg whites until it forms stiff peaks.
2. Second bowl: Blend the egg yolks, coconut flour, sweetener, and cooking powder.
3. Add the melted butter little by little; mixing to make sure it is a smooth uniformity.
4. Add the dairy and vanilla, blend well.
5. Delicately fold spoons of the whisked egg whites into the yolk mixture.
6. Place enough of the waffle mix into the warm waffle machine to make one waffle. Make until golden.

7. Duplicate until all the mix has been used.

Lunch: Chipotle Pulled Pork Lettuce Wraps with Avocado Aioli

Prep + Cooking time: 15 minutes

Servings: 2

Ingredients:

For the Avocado Aioli

- 1/2 of an Avocado
- 2 Tablespoons of entire 30 Mayonnaise
- 1 Lime, juiced
- 1 Garlic clove, finely minced
- Sodium & Pepper, to taste
- Water, for thinning if required

For the Lettuce Wraps

- 1 Butter Lettuce, scattered into lettuce cups
- 2 Mugs of warm Chipotle Pulled Pork
- 1 slice of Avocado
- Lime Wedges and Cilantro

Directions:

1. Crush the avocado and whisk in the mayo, lime drink, garlic, sodium, and pepper.
2. Pile the pork into the lettuce mugs, top with chopped up avocado, drizzle with the aioli and top with cilantro and lime.

Dinner: Buffalo Chicken Jalapeno Popper Casserole

Prep + Cooking time: 45 minutes

Servings: 4

Ingredients

- 6 small Rooster Thighs
- 6 pieces Bacon
- 3 medium Jalapenos
- 12 oz. Cream Cheese
- 1/4 glass Mayonnaise
- 4 oz. Shredded Cheddar
- 2 oz. Shredded Mozzarella Cheese
- 1/4 glass Frank's Red Hot
- Sodium and Pepper to Taste

Directions:

1. De-bone all poultry thighs and pre-heat oven to 400F. Bake fowl thighs for 40 minutes at 400F.
2. Chop 6 pieces of bacon into bits and place into a skillet over medium warmth. Once bacon is crisped, add jalapenos into the pan.
3. Once peppers are tender and grilled, add cream parmesan cheese, mayo, and frank's red hot to the skillet. Mix alongside one another and season to taste.
4. Remove chicken breast from the oven and let cool just a little. After they are cold enough, take away the skins from the rooster.
5. Lay hen into a casserole dish, then pass on cream cheese concoction over it, then top with cheddar and mozzarella parmesan cheese.

6. Bake for 10-15 minutes at 400F. Broil for 3-5 minutes to complete.

DAY 3

Breakfast: Keto Taco Breakfast Time Skillet

Prep + Cooking time: 15 minutes

Servings: 6

Ingredients:

- 1 pound beef
- 4 tablespoons Taco Seasoning
- 2/3 glass of water
- 10 large eggs
- 1 1/2 mugs shredded razor-sharp cheddar mozzarella cheese, divided
- 1/4 heavy glass cream
- 1 Roma tomato, diced
- 1 medium avocado, peeled, pitted and cubed
- 1/4 cup sliced up black olives
- 2 renewable onions, sliced
- 1/4 glass sour cream
- 1/4 glass salsa
- 1 jalapeno, sliced up (optional)
- 2 tablespoons torn fresh cilantro (optional)

Directions:

1. Brown the beef in a sizable skillet over medium-high heating.
2. Mix in the taco seasoning and water. Reduce the high temperature to low and let simmer until sauce has thickened and covered the meats.

3. Remove half of the seasoned beef after 5 minutes from the skillet and reserve.

4. Split the eggs into a huge mixing dish and whisk. Add 1 glass of the cheddar cheese, and cream to the eggs and whisk.

5. Preheat the oven to 375°F.

6. Pour the egg mixture over the surface of the meat and mix. Bake for thirty minutes.

7. Top with the other beef left, 1/2 cup of cheddar cheese, tomato, avocado, olives, onion, sour cream, and salsa. Garnish with jalapeno and cilantro.

Lunch: Grilled Lemon Natural Herb Mediterranean Poultry Salad

Prep + Cooking time: 10 minutes

Servings: 4

Ingredients:

Marinade/Dressing

- 2 tablespoons essential olive oil
- 1/4 glass fresh squeezed lemon drink
- 2 tablespoons of water
- 2 tablespoons of burgundy or merlot wine vinegar
- 2 tablespoons of fresh cut parsley
- 2 teaspoons of dried out basil
- 2 teaspoons of garlic clove, minced
- 1 teaspoon of dried out oregano
- 1 teaspoon of salt
- Pepper, to taste
- 500 g of 4 skinless, boneless fowl thigh fillets

Salad

- 4 mugs of Romaine (or Cos) lettuce leaves
- 1 large cucumber, diced
- 2 Roma tomato vegetables, diced
- 1 red onion, sliced
- 1 avocado, sliced
- Lemon wedges, to serve

Directions:

1. Whisk together the marinade in a huge jug. Pour out half of the marinade into a big, shallow dish. Refrigerate for future use.

2. Marinade chicken for 15-30 minutes. Put together all the salad materials and combination in a sizable salad bowl.

3. Once poultry is ready, warm 1 tablespoon of olive oil in a barbeque grill skillet or a barbeque grill dish over medium-high heating. Grill rooster on both edges until browned and thoroughly cooked.

4. Allow chicken to relax for five minutes; cut and pour over salad. Serve with lemon wedges.

Dinner: Thai Bbq Pork Salad

Prep + Cooking time: 15 minutes

Servings: 2

Ingredients

The Salad

- 10 oz . pulled pork
- 2 mugs romaine lettuce
- 1/4 cup sliced cilantro
- 1/4 medium red bell pepper, chopped

The Sauce

- 2 tablespoons tomato paste
- 8 teaspoons soy sauce
- 1 tablespoons creamy peanut
- 2 tablespoons sliced cilantro
- 1/2 cup of lime juice
- 1 teaspoon five spice
- 1 teaspoon red curry paste
- teaspoon rice wines vinegar
- 1/4 teaspoon red pepper flakes
- 1 teaspoon seafood sauce
- 10 drops liquid stevia
- 1/2 teaspoon mango extract

Direction:

1. In a dish, incorporate all the sauce substances together (aside from cilantro and lime zest).

2. Chop cilantro and lime and enhance the sauce.

3. Mix the Thai BBQ sauce together, and then reserve.

4. Using your hands, or a blade, pull aside the pork.

5. Serve your salad, pork, and sauce.

DAY 4

Breakfast: Paleo Strawberry Granola

Prep + Cooking time: 5 minutes

Servings: 1-2

Ingredients:

- 6-7 washed, cut strawberries
- 1-2 Tablespoon of chocolates
- 1-2 Tablespoon of favorite raw Nuts

Directions:

1. Clean and chop your strawberries and add them to the bowl.
2. Add your delicious chocolate + nut products.
3. Add a tiny spritz of lemon drink, mix everything up and either add straight away or store in the refrigerator.

Lunch: California Turkey and Bacon Lettuce Wraps With Basil-Mayo

Prep + Cooking time: 5 minutes

Servings: 2

Ingredients:

- 1 head iceberg lettuce
- 4 pieces gluten-free deli turkey
- 4 slices gluten-free bacon, cooked properly
- 1 avocado, thinly sliced
- 1 Roma tomato, thinly sliced

For the Basil-Mayo

- 1/2 glass gluten-free mayonnaise
- 6 large basil leaves, torn
- 1 teaspoon lemon juice
- 1 garlic clove, chopped
- Table salt
- Pepper

Directions:

1. For the Basil-Mayo: incorporate ingredients in a tiny food processor chip then process until clean.
2. Construct two large lettuce leaves then level on 1 cut of turkey and slather with Basil-Mayo. Level on another cut of turkey accompanied by the bacon, and some pieces of

both avocado and tomato. Season softly with sodium and pepper then collapse underneath up, the sides in, and move just like a burrito. Slice in two and serve cold.

Dinner: Keto Salmon Curry

Prep + Cooking time: 35 minutes

Servings: 2

Ingredients:

- 1/2 medium onion, diced or finely chopped
- 2 mugs green beans, diced
- 10g curry powder
- 1 teaspoon garlic clove powder
- Coconut milk
- 2 cups bone broth
- 1 lb of fresh salmon, diced
- 2 Tablespoons (30 ml) coconut olive oil
- Sodium and pepper, to taste
- 2 Tablespoons basil (4 g), cut, for garnish

Directions:

1. Heat the diced onion in the coconut oil until translucent.
2. Add the green coffee beans and saute for a few seconds more.
3. Add the broth or drinking water and bring to a boil.
4. Add the natural curry powder, natural garlic powder, and salmon.
5. Add the coconut cream and simmer before salmon is prepared (3-5 minutes).
6. Add sodium and pepper to flavor and serve with the cut basil.

DAY 5

Breakfast: One Minute English Muffins

Prep + Cooking time: 1 minute

Servings: 2

Ingredients:

- 1 1/2 teaspoons coconut essential oil
- 1 1/2 tablespoons almond butter
- 1 egg
- 1 tablespoon coconut flour
- 1/4 teaspoon cooking powder
- 1/8 teaspoon salt

Directions:

1. Stir coconut olive oil, almond butter, and egg until well put together.
2. Blend in coconut flour, cooking powder and sodium.
3. Microwave on high temperature for 1 minute.
4. Take away the muffin from the glass and slice in two.

Lunch: Cheddar-Wrapped Taco Rolls

Prep + Cooking time: 22 minute

Serves 3

Ingredients:

For the crust

- 2 cups of cheddar cheese

For the toppings

- 1 cup taco meat (cooked and seasoned ahead of time)
- 1/4 cup tomatoes, chopped
- 1/2 of an avocado, diced
- 2 teaspoon of Sriracha mayo or taco sauce

Directions:

1. Preheat oven to 400F.
2. Cover a little baking sheet with parchment paper.
3. Grease the parchment paper lightly.
4. Sprinkle shredded cheddar cheese to cover the baking sheet with one layer.
5. Bake for about 15 minutes.
6. Add taco meat and cook for 5-10 minutes.
7. Remove from oven and baking pan by holding the sides of the parchment paper.
8. Add the cold toppings in a single layer.
9. Use a pizza cutter to slice top to bottom and make 3-4 slices.

Dinner: Baked Halibut with Lemon & Thai Chili

Prep + Cooking time: 25 minutes

Servings: 4

Ingredients:

- 4 mugs spinach, packed
- 2 11oz halibut steaks, about an inch thick
- Juice of half of a lemon
- Sodium and pepper to taste
- A sprinkle with smoked paprika
- 1/2 lemon, chopped up into 4
- Green onions, sliced
- 1 red Thai chili, deseeded, halved & sliced up thinly
- 1 cup cherry tomato vegetables, halved
- 2 tablespoon of avocado oil, divided

Directions:

1. Preheat oven to 400F.
2. Lay two bits of halibut together with each pile of spinach.
3. Squash the lemon drink on the fillets, season to style with smoked paprika and top each one with a cut of lemon.
4. Divide the sliced up green onions, Thai chili, and cherry tomato vegetables equally between your two squares. Split the avocado oil so that all piece of seafood is topped with about 1/2 tablespoon of oil.

5. Cover the foil around the fish firmly & place both deals on a cooking tray.

6. Bake for about quarter-hour, until fish is grilled through and flakes easily.

7. Remove the fish and dish, spooning the juices on the fillets before serving.

DAY 6

Breakfast: Fudge Keto Overnight Oats

Prep + Cooking time: 1 hour

Servings: 2

Ingredients:

- 2/3 glass (160 ml) full-fat coconut dairy
- 1/2 glass (75 grams) Manitoba Harvest Hemp Hearts
- 2 tablespoons of cacao powder
- 1 tablespoon of sunflower butter
- 1 tablespoon chia seed
- 3-4 drops of liquid stevia
- 1/2 teaspoon vanilla extract
- pinch finely surface Himalayan rock and roll salt

Directions:

1. Add all elements to a 350 ml, or much larger pot with a cover. Stir until blended.
2. Place overnight in the fridge for at least 8 hours.
3. The next day, add new dairy until satisfied.
4. Separate between two small bowls, add toppings if desired.

Lunch: Vegetarian Keto Club Salad

Prep + Cooking time: 15 minutes

Servings: 3

Ingredients:

- 2 tablespoons sour cream
- 2 tablespoons mayonnaise
- 1/2 teaspoon of garlic powder
- 1/2 teaspoon of onion powder
- 1 teaspoon of dried parsley
- 1 tablespoon milk
- 3 large hard-boiled eggs, sliced
- 4 ounces cheddar cheese, cubed
- 3 cups romaine lettuce, torn into pieces
- 1/2 cup cherry tomatoes, halved
- 1 cup diced cucumber
- 1 tablespoon dijon mustard

Directions:

1. Mix the sour cream, mayonnaise, and dried herbs together.
2. Mix with one tablespoon of milk. Keep adding milk till you are satisfied with the texture.
3. Include fresh veggies, cheese, and sliced egg to your salad.
4. Add to the center 1 tablespoon Dijon mustard.
5. Sprinkle with the prepared dressing, about 2 tablespoons for one serving.

Dinner: Oven Fried Tilapia

Prep + Cooking time: 15 minutes

Servings: 4

Ingredients:

- 4 filets Tilapia (~1 lb.)
- 1/4 glass Mayonnaise
- 3 tablespoon of Parmesan Cheese
- 3 tablespoon of Pork Dust Particles
- 1 tablespoon of Lemon Juice
- 2 teaspoon of Minced Garlic
- 1 handful Fresh Basil, chopped
- Sodium and Pepper to Taste

Directions:

1. Pre-heat oven to 400F.
2. Brand a 9x9 cooking skillet with foil and lay down the fish within the pan.
3. Season tilapia with sodium, pepper, lemon drink, garlic clove, and fresh basil.
4. Spread mayonnaise over the fish, then sprinkle parmesan cheese and pork particles also.
5. Bake for 16-18 minutes or until tilapia is adequately cooked through.

DAY 7

Breakfast: Oven Cooked Eggs Recipe

Prep + Cooking time: 15 minutes

Servings: 4-6

Ingredients:

- 1 Dozen Eggs
- Sodium and Pepper to taste
- Nonstick Food preparation Spray

Directions:

1. Preheat oven to 350F.
2. Split eggs into a gently greased muffin tin. Sprinkle little sodium and pepper onto the eggs.
3. Bake at 350F for 15 minutes.
4. Remove from oven. Refrigerate for four days.

Lunch: Salmon & Avocado Nori Rolls

Prep + Cooking time: 10 minutes

Serves: 1

Ingredients:

- 3 square nori sheets (seaweed wrappers)
- 150-180 g / 5-6 oz cooked salmon or tinned salmon
- 1/3 of red pepper, sliced into thin strips
- 1/2 avocado, sliced into strips
- 1/2 small cucumber, sliced into strips
- 1 spring onion/scallion, cut into 2-3" pieces
- 2 tablespoons mayonnaise
- 1 tablespoon hot sauce or Sriracha sauce
- 1 teaspoon black or white sesame seeds
- Coconut aminos for dipping, optional

Directions:

1. Lay the nori sheet on a flat surface.
2. Add a third of the salmon to the nori sheet and top with pepper, cucumber, and avocado strips.
3. Add some green onion, mayonnaise, and hot sauce. Sprinkle the cut rolls with sesame seeds.
4. Lay the roll on the cutting board and cut into bite-size pieces.
5. Serve straight away with some coconut aminos or extra mayo for dipping.

Dinner: Cumin Spiced Meat Wraps

Prep + cooking time: 25 mins

Serves: 2

Ingredients

- 1-2 tablespoon of coconut oil
- 1/4 onion, diced small
- 2/3 lb surface beef
- 1 red bell pepper, diced small
- 2 tablespoon of cilantro, chopped
- 1 teaspoon of ginger, minced
- 4 cloves garlic, minced
- 2 teaspoon of cumin
- Sodium and pepper, to taste
- 8 large cabbage leaves

Directions:

1. Place 1-2 tablespoon of coconut oil into a frying skillet and saute the onions, meat, and peppers on medium temperature.
2. When the bottom beef is prepared, add the cilantro, ginger, garlic clove, cumin, sodium, and pepper to style.
3. Fill a sizable container 3/4 full with water and to boil.
4. Using tongs, put each cabbage leaf in the boiling water. Then plunge each leaf into some cold water before draining and inserting into a dish.
5. Spoon the meat blend onto each lettuce leaf and fold.

DAY 8

Breakfast: Avocado and Salmon Low Carbohydrate Breakfast

Prep + Cooking time: 10 minutes

Serves: 2

Ingredients:

- 1 ripe organic and natural avocado (about 100 grams or 2.5 oz)
- 60 grams of smoked salmon
- 30 grams of fresh goat cheese
- 2 tablespoons of organic and natural extra virgin olive oil
- 1 lemon juice
- a pinch of sea salt

Directions:

1. Slice the avocado in two and take away the seed.
2. In a tiny food processor combine all of those other ingredients until coarsely cut.
3. Place the cream inside the avocado.
4. Serve immediately.

Lunch: Caprese Tuna Salad Stuffed Tomatoes

Prep + Cooking time: 10 minutes

Serves: 1

Ingredients:

- 1 medium tomato
- 1 (5oz) of Can tuna
- 2 tablespoon of balsamic vinegar
- 1 tablespoon of sliced mozzarella
- 1 tablespoon of sliced fresh basil
- 1 tablespoon of chopped green onion

Directions:

1. Slice the top 1/4-inch from the tomato. Scoop out the insides of the tomato.
2. Stir the drained tuna, balsamic vinegar, mozzarella, basil, and green onion together.
3. Pour the tuna salad in the hollowed out tomato, and enjoy!

Dinner: Cauliflower Crusted Grilled Mozzarella Cheese Sandwiches

Prep + Cooking time: 45 minutes

Servings: 2

Ingredients:

- 1 medium cauliflower (fresh)
- 1 large egg
- 1/2 glass shredded Parmesan cheese
- 1 teaspoon of Italian supplement seasoning
- 2 thick pieces of white cheddar mozzarella cheese

Directions:

1. Preheat oven to 450F.
2. Crush the cauliflower and place it in large microwave safe dish and microwave for 2 minutes.
3. Stir to mix the cauliflower. Place back to the microwave and make for another three minutes.
4. Remove and blend again so that the cauliflower cooks equally.
5. Place back to microwave and make for five minutes.
6. Allow cauliflower to cool for a few seconds. Then add egg and mozzarella cheese.
7. Bake cauliflower for approximately 15-18 minutes or until darkish.
8. Put together with your sandwiches and serve.

DAY 9

Breakfast: Fluffy Scrambled Cinnamon Pancakes

Prep + Cooking time: 15 minutes

Servings: 4

Ingredients:

- 8 large eggs
- 8 oz cream mozzarella cheese
- 2 tbsp heavy cream
- 8 pieces of bacon
- Cinnamon Vanilla
- coconut olive oil or ghee
- salted butter
- sugar-free syrup (optional)
- strawberries (optional)

Directions:

1. Blend all ingredients smoothly together.
2. Heat a medium frying skillet.
3. Add 1 tablespoon coconut essential oil or ghee.
4. Once hot, add your pancake combination.
5. Make for just a few minutes then stir.
6. Once every one of the egg is ready, put each into four bowls.

Lunch: Avocado Egg Salad

Prep + Cooking time: 15 minutes

Servings: 4

Ingredients:

- 4 large hard-boiled eggs
- 1 avocado, diced
- 2 green onions, chopped up into skinny rounds
- 4 pieces of low-sodium bacon, prepared to a desired clean and crumbled
- 1/4- glass nonfat natural yogurt
- 1 tablespoon zero fat sour cream
- 1 complete lime, juiced
- 1 tablespoon of snipped fresh dill
- 1/4 teaspoon salt
- 1/8 teaspoon fresh floor pepper
- dill and crumbled bacon, for garnish (optional)

Directions:

1. Boil eggs in the oven for thirty minutes at 325F.
2. Peel off eggshell and dice.
3. Inside a salad bowl, incorporate diced eggs, avocado, green onions, and bacon.
4. Inside a mixing dish, whisk yogurt, sour cream, lime drink, dill, sodium, and pepper; whisk until well merged.
5. Add yogurt mixture to the egg salad.
6. Garnish with dill and crumbled bacon.
7. Serve.

Dinner: Stuffed Pork Chops

Prep + Cooking time: 1hr 13 minutes

Servings: 4

Ingredients:

- 4 Thick Pork Chops
- 3 Pieces Bacon
- 3 Oz. Bleu Cheese
- 3 Oz. Feta Cheese
- 60 g Green Onion
- 2 Oz. Cream Cheese
- Sodium, pepper, and garlic clove natural powder to taste

Directions:

1. Make the bacon in a skillet, reserve the grease and place the bacon aside.
2. Combine the Bleu and feta cheeses in a bowl.
3. Mix the bacon and green onions.
4. Add the cream parmesan cheese.
5. Slice open up the pork chops and pour the parmesan cheese mixture.
6. Apply sodium, pepper, and garlic clove powder to the pork chops.
7. Over high temperature, with bacon grease in the skillet, sear for 5 minutes.
8. Pour chops into a greased skillet and cook at 350 degrees for 55 minutes.
9. Remove pork chops and let leftovers three minutes before serving.

DAY 10

Breakfast: Ultimate Breakfast Time Roll-Ups

Prep + Cooking time: 30 minutes

Servings: 5

Ingredients:

- 10 large eggs
- Sodium and pepper to taste
- 1.5 mugs shredded cheddar cheese
- 5 pieces bacon, cooked
- 5 patties breakfast time sausage, cooked

Directions:

1. Pre-heat a nonstick skillet over medium-high warmth.
2. After the skillet is hot add the whisked eggs at a medium temperature. Season the eggs with sodium and pepper.
3. Cover and leave to prepare for a few moments before the egg is grilled all through.
4. Sprinkle about 1/3 glass of cheese all around the egg. Cut a part of bacon, then break a sausage patty in two and place that down at the top.
5. Carefully spin the egg in the fillings.
6. Serve

Lunch: Fresh Tuna Salad Recipe

Prep + Cooking time: 10 minutes

Servings: 1-2

Ingredients:

- 1 can of tuna
- 1 Roma tomato, diced
- 1 Persian cucumber, diced
- 1/4 of a tiny crimson onion, chopped
- 1 tablespoon of mayo
- 1 tablespoon of ketchup
- Fine sea salt to flavor

Directions:

1. In a very medium size dish, add every one of the ingredients and mix.
2. Serve with chopped up cucumbers; potato chips made without natural veg oils.

Dinner: Coffee Infused Ribeye Steak

Prep + Cooking time: 10 minutes

Servings: 2

Ingredients:

- 1 Ribeye Steak (~12 oz.)
- 1 tsp. Jacobsen Stumptown Espresso Sodium (per pound steak)

Directions:

1. Ready the steak by using a reverse sear method.
2. Once rested, cut steak and dish.
3. Finish steak with a large part of Jacobsen Stumptown Coffee Salt.

DAY 11

Breakfast: Keto Burrito Bowl

Prep + Cooking time: 20 minutes

Servings: 2

Ingredients:

- 1/2 pound trim ground beef
- 1 tablespoon of keto taco seasoning
- 3/4 glass water
- 1/3 cauliflower riced
- 2 tablespoon of cilantro chopped
- 1 tablespoon of ghee
- 3 eggs beaten
- sea sodium & pepper to taste

Directions:

1. In a large skillet, brown surface meat and remove any unwanted fat that makes as it cooks.
2. Add your keto taco seasoning and boil for a few moments.
3. Mix the taco meats, riced cauliflower, cilantro, and salt together.
4. Make the cauliflower for three to four 4 minutes, and then press it aside to make space for the scrambled egg.
5. Melt ghee and put in the beaten egg.
6. Whisk the egg and shake the skillet as it cooks to split up the curd.
7. After the egg scrambles to your preference, mix it within the already prepared dish.

8. Season with salt and pepper to flavor.

Lunch: Spicy Thai Rooster Zoodle Soup

Prep + Cooking time: 30 minutes

Servings: 4

Ingredients:

- 1 Tablespoon Coconut Oil
- 2 Chicken Breasts
- Salt & Pepper
- 2 Mugs Fresh Snow Peas
- 1 Teaspoon Freshly Grated Ginger
- 3 Garlic clove Cloves, finely minced
- 5 Scallions, very thinly sliced
- 4 Cups Hen Stock
- 2 Teaspoons Green Curry Paste
- 1 Dried out Thai Chili
- 1 Medium Zucchini
- 1 Medium Yellow Squash
- Peppers, for garnish

Directions

1. Heat the essential coconut oil over medium-high warmth.
2. Season the chicken parts liberally with sodium and pepper and add these to the hot skillet. Leave the chicken to cook for just a few minutes and then start moving it around the pan. Add the snow peas and saute for only a few minutes until it's crisp-tender.
3. Remove and reserve.

4. Add the ginger, garlic clove, and scallions to the skillet and saute for 30 sec. Pour in the chicken breast stock and then mix in the green curry paste. Add the Thai chili and bring the broth to a minimal simmer for approximately 10 minutes.

5. To put together the bowls, begin by placing a small number of both zucchini and squash noodles into the soup dish. Top with a few of the rooster/snow pea concoction. Ladle a few of the broth over the top.

6. Garnish the soup with additional scallions and red bell pepper. Enjoy!

Dinner: Keto Butter Chicken

Prep + Cooking time: 30 minutes

Servings: 6

Ingredients:

- 1.5 lbs chicken white meat
- 2 Tablespoons garam masala
- 3 teaspoons ginger, grated
- 3 teaspoons garlic clove, minced
- 4 oz natural yogurt
- 1 tablespoon coconut oil

sauce

- 2 tablespoons ghee
- 1 onion
- 2 teaspoons ginger, grated
- 2 teaspoons garlic clove, minced
- 14.5 oz smashed tomatoes
- 1 teaspoon chili powder
- 1 tablespoon coriander
- 2 teaspoons cumin
- 1/2 glass of heavy cream
- 1/2 tablespoon of garam masala

optional:

- cilantro

- cauliflower rice

Directions:

1. Cut hen into 2 inches pieces and place in a huge bowl with 2 tablespoons garam masala, 1 teaspoon grated ginger, and 1 teaspoon minced garlic. Add the yogurt, mix to mix. Chill at least thirty minutes.

2. For the sauce, place the onion, ginger, garlic clove, crushed tomato vegetables and spices in a blender, and mix until smooth. Reserve.

3. Heat 1 tablespoon of oil in a sizable skillet over medium-high heat. Place the chicken in the skillet, browning three to four minutes per part. Once browned pour in the sauce and leave for 5 to 6 minutes much longer.

4. Mix in the heavy cream and ghee, continue steadily for another minute. Top with cilantro, and provide with cauliflower grain if desired.

DAY 12

Breakfast: Keto Mexican Breakfast Time Casserole

Prep + Cooking time: 30 minutes

Servings: 6

Ingredients:

- 1 lb thick-cut bacon (450 g)
- 2 tablespoon of reserved bacon grease or ghee (30 ml)
- 1 small turnip, diced (300 g/ 10.6 oz)
- 1 large red onion, thinly sliced up (150 g/ 5.3 oz)
- 3 mugs spinach (90 g/ 3.2 oz)
- 12 large eggs
- 1/3 cup dairy (80 ml/ 2.7 fl oz)
- 1 tablespoon of salt
- 1 tablespoon of garlic clove powder
- 1/2 tablespoon of dark pepper
- 1/2 glass of shredded cheddar cheese (57 g/ 2 oz)

Directions:

1. Preheat the oven to 400F. Slice the bacon into 2-inches pieces and arrange over a parchment lined baking sheet.
2. Bake for quarter-hour until clean.
3. Heat the reserved bacon minimally in a medium skillet.
4. Add the turnip and onion, prepare for about 5-7 minutes.
5. Top the turnip and onion with the spinach.

6. Whisk the eggs, dairy, and spices.

7. Sprinkle the mozzarella cheese and organize the bacon in one layer over the surface of the casserole.

8. Place it in the oven and bake 20-25 minutes or before eggs are placed.

9. Store and keep refrigerated for 5 days and nights.

Lunch: Fresh Sriracha Broccoli Salad Keto

Prep + Cooking time: 20 minutes

Servings: 4

Ingredients:

- 4 heaping cups sliced broccoli
- 1/2 red bell pepper
- 1 cup mayonnaise
- 1/2 glass shredded cheddar cheese
- 1/4 cup dried roasted salted sunflower seed products (shelled)
- 6 pieces of bacon
- 1/2 tablespoon of apple cider vinegar
- 1/4 to 1/2 tablespoon of sriracha sauce (depending on your desired spice)
- salt and newly cracked dark-colored pepper to taste

Directions:

1. Mix all materials collectively in a dish and toss.
2. Store in a closed pot for at least two minutes, then enjoy!

Dinner: Taco Stuffed Avocados

Prep + Cooking time: 20 minutes

Servings: 6

Ingredients:

- 1 pound surface beef
- 1 tablespoon Chili Powder
- 1/2 teaspoon Salt
- 3/4 teaspoon Cumin
- 1/2 teaspoon Dried out Oregano
- 1/4 teaspoon Garlic clove Powder
- 1/4 teaspoon Onion Powder
- 4 oz. tomato sauce
- 3 avocados halved
- 1 glass shredded cheddar cheese
- 1/4 glass cherry tomato vegetables sliced
- 1/4 glass lettuce shredded

Additional toppings:

- cilantro
- sour cream

Directions:

1. Cook meat in a medium high temperature.
2. Add the seasonings and the tomato sauce. Make for approximately 3-4 minutes.

3. Take away the pit from the halved avocados. Fill the crater with the taco beef. Top with mozzarella cheese, tomato vegetables, lettuce, cilantro and sour cream.

DAY 13

Breakfast: 1 Minute Keto Muffin

Prep + Cooking time: 1 minute

Servings: 1

Ingredients:

- 1 large egg
- 2 tsp coconut flour
- pinch cooking soda
- pinch salt

Directions:

1. Grease a ramekin dish with coconut engine oil or butter.
2. In the mug, merge all the materials as well as a fork to make sure it is lump free.
3. Place the 1-minute keto muffin dough in the greased ramekin and make meals in the microwave on high for 1 minute. On the other hand, they could be baked in an oven, at 200C/400F for 12 minutes.
4. Cut in two and serve.

Lunch: Low Carbohydrate Vietnamese Noodle Dish Salad

Prep + Cooking time: 45 minutes

Servings: 4

Ingredients:

The Salad

- 2 Shirataki Noodles
- 1 pound Boneless Country Style Pork Ribs
- 1/4 pound Shrimp butterflied
- 1/8 glass Sprouted Mung Beans
- Salt to taste
- 4 mugs Romaine Lettuce chopped
- 1-ounce Peanuts chopped
- 1/2 glass Cucumber julienned
- 9 sprigs Cilantro

The Dressing

- 1/4 glass Water
- 2 tablespoons White Grain Vinegar
- 1/4 glass Red Boat Seafood Sauce
- 2 tablespoons Erythritol
- 1 tablespoon Thai Garlic clove Chili Sauce

Directions:

The Salad

1. Boil shirataki noodles for a few minutes.

2. Drain the noodles and chill in refrigerator until prepared to add the salad.

3. Salt the pork to your taste.

4. Barbeque grill pork and shrimp over high temperature. Reserve once appropriately cooked through.

5. To create the salad, separate each prepped salad element into four parts to spread into four independent bowls. The bowls should be large enough to permit tossing and mixing up.

6. Layer romaine, grilled and chilled shirataki noodles, roasted pork and shrimp, mung coffee beans, cucumber, cilantro, and peanuts.

The Dressing

1. Whisk together water, white grain vinegar, seafood sauce, erythritol, and Thai garlic clove chili sauce.

2. Serve drizzled on the noodle salad, then toss salad to distribute consistently.

Dinner: Cheeseburger Calzone

Prep + Cooking time: 45 minutes

Servings: 8

Ingredients:

- 1.5lb 85/15 earth beef
- 1/2c yellowish onion, diced
- 4 strips thick trim bacon
- 4 dill pickle spears
- 8oz cream mozzarella cheese, separated
- 1c shredded cheddar cheese
- 1/2c mayonnaise
- 1c shredded mozzarella cheese
- 1c almond flour
- 1 egg

Directions:

1. Pre-heat the oven to 425F.
2. Make the pizza crust by combining the mozzarella cheese and 4 oz . of cream cheese together; microwave about 35 secs until the parmesan cheese melt. Add the almond flour and egg to the parmesan cheese and blend until it forms a dough; reserve.
3. Over medium warmth, cook the bottom meat until browned.
4. Make the bacon in your selected method. Let cool, break right into small parts and reserve.
5. Dice the yellowish onion; enhance the ground meat until softened.
6. Chop the dill pickle spears.

7. Add the bacon, pickles, 4 oz . of cream cheese, mayonnaise and cheddar cheese to the bottom beef. Mix until all cheeses are melted and thoroughly incorporated.

8. Spin out the dough over a parchment-lined cooking sheet.

9. Spoon the cheeseburger concoction into the middle of the dough.

10. Collapse up and take the ends over into the center so that it is closed.

11. Bake about a quarter-hour until golden brownish. Let sit ten minutes before cutting.

DAY 14

Breakfast: Bacon Burger Breakfast Time Hash

Prep + Cooking time: 25 minutes

Servings: 4

Ingredients:

- 8oz Applegate Naturals
- 4 cups of sugary potatoes, peeled & grated
- 2 garlic cloves, minced
- 1/2 cup of diced onion
- 1/2 pound of grass-fed beef
- 4 free range eggs
- 1/4 cup sliced green onions

Directions:

1. Heat your oven to about 400 degrees.
2. Fry bacon until crispy.
3. Remove bacon and chop into small bits.
4. Add the shredded potatoes to the skillet with the rest of the bacon grease.
5. Prepare for 2-3 minutes then blend and leave for another 2-3 minutes.
6. Prepare garlic clove and onions until onions are translucent.
7. Add the beef and prepare until fully brownish and crumbly.
8. Place potatoes and some portion of the bacon back to the pan.
9. Mix all the ingredients jointly then create four pieces into the oven, and split an egg into each piece.

10. Sprinkle with leftover bacon and place skillet into the oven for 12 minutes or until your yolks are done.
11. Remove from the oven and add green onions before you serve.

Lunch: Cheeseburger Lettuce Wraps

Prep + Cooking time: 23 minutes

Servings: 3

Ingredients:

- 2 pounds lean earth beef
- 1/2 teaspoon seasoned salt
- 1 teaspoon dark pepper
- 1 teaspoon dried out oregano
- 6 slices American cheese
- 2 large romaine lettuce, rinsed then dried
- 2 tomatoes, sliced up thin
- small red onion, chopped up thin

Spread

- 1/4 glass light mayo
- 3 Tablespoons ketchup
- 1 Tablespoon dill pickle relish
- dash of sodium and pepper

Directions:

1. Heat a barbeque grill or skillet on medium temperature.
2. In a sizable bowl, mix alongside one another ground meat, seasoned sodium, pepper, and oregano.
3. Divide mix into 6 parts then spins each into a ball. Press each ball down even to create a patty.

4. Place patties on barbeque grill/pan and make meals for about 4 minutes on each part or until grilled to your preference. (If by using a skillet, only prepare 3 at the same time to avoid over-crowding).

5. Place a cup of cheese on each grilled burger. Place each burger on a sizable little bit of lettuce. Top with the spread, one cut tomato, red onion and other things that you like. Cover the lettuce up and serve.

Dinner: One Skillet Balsamic Chicken And Veggies

Prep + Cooking time: 1hr 30 minutes

Servings: 4

Ingredients:

- 6 tablespoons balsamic vinegar
- 1/2 glass zesty Italian dressing
- 1.25 pounds poultry tenders (or chest)
- 2 heads broccoli
- 1 glass baby carrots
- 1/2 pint cherry tomatoes
- 1 teaspoon Italian seasoning
- 3 tablespoons essential olive oil
- 1/2 teaspoon garlic clove powder

Optional: fresh parsley, sodium, and pepper

Directions:

1. Preheat the oven to 400F.
2. Whisk along the balsamic vinegar and zesty Italian dressing.
3. Add the poultry tenders. Marinate for at least thirty minutes.
4. Chop the broccoli into small portions. Cut the baby carrots in two.
5. Place broccoli + carrots on the ready holder with the cherry tomato vegetables, Italian seasoning, essential olive oil, natural garlic powder, and then add seasoned sodium and pepper to style.
6. Roast the vegetables for 10-15 minutes.

7. Remove from the oven and turn around. Section the vegetables to each aspect of the holder and place the chicken breast tenders (discard marinade) in the guts. Brush 1/3 glass of the balsamic + Italian concoction over the poultry.

8. Go back to the oven and make for another 7-15 minutes depending on the size of your fowl. Serve the poultry and vegetables with the rest of the Balsamic + Italian concoction. Top with newly sliced parsley if desired.

DAY 15

Breakfast: Healthy Flourless Cinnamon Bun Breakfast Time Doughnuts

Prep + Cooking time: 30 minutes

Servings: 4

Ingredients:

- 3/4 glass of coconut flour, sifted
- 1 glass of almond flour, filtered
- 1/2 tablespoon of cooking soda
- 1 teaspoon of cinnamon
- 4 large eggs
- 1/2 cup of milk
- 3 teaspoon of drippy almond butter
- 1/2 glass of honey

Directions:

1. Preheat the oven to 350 degrees.
2. Add the dried up ingredients and combine well.
3. Whisk the dairy and eggs alongside one another.
4. In another dish, melt your nut butter with honey and incorporate both into the dry mixture. Mix until an extremely dense batter is shaped.
5. Pour into a greased doughnut skillet and bake for 25-30 minutes, or until prepared through.
6. Remove from oven and let be seated for five minutes before moving to an air conditioning rack. Keep it frost once cooled.

Lunch: Zucchini Pizza Boats

Prep + Cooking time: 15 minutes

Servings: 6

Ingredients:

- 6 small zucchini (2 1/2 pounds)
- 1 tablespoon of essential olive oil
- 1 clove garlic clove , finely minced
- Salt and newly ground dark pepper
- 1 glass marinara sauce
- 1 1/2 mugs shredded mozzarella cheese (6 oz)
- 1/3 glass finely shredded parmesan mozzarella cheese (1.4 oz)
- 1/2 cup minuscule pepperoni slices
- 2 tablespoon of cut fresh oregano

Directions:

1. Preheat oven to 400 degrees.
2. Slice each zucchini into halves
3. Align on the well-prepared baking sheet.
4. Sprinkle with sodium and pepper to flavor then brush with about 1 tablespoon of marinara sauce over each zucchini.
5. Sprinkle tops consistently with mozzarella cheese then with parmesan cheese. Top with pepperoni pieces
6. Bake in preheated oven for about 12 - 18 minutes on.
7. Remove from oven and sprinkle with cut fresh oregano. Serve warm.

Dinner: One Pan Lemon Garlic Baked Salmon + Asparagus

Prep + Cooking time: 10 minutes

Servings: 6

Ingredients:

- 4 - 6 oz or 170 g salmon fillets, skin removed
- 2 tablespoons minced garlic
- 2 tablespoons fresh chopped parsley
- 1/3 cup of lemon juice
- Olive oil cooking spray
- 1 teaspoon Kosher salt
- 1/2 teaspoon cracked black pepper
- 4 bunches asparagus
- 1 lemon, sliced to garnish
- 1/3 cup beans/peas or any other greens

Directions:

1. Preheat oven grill to high heat.
2. Put the salmon fillet on a tray
3. Coat with garlic and parsley; pour lemon juice and spray with olive oil. Arrange the asparagus and greens around the salmon in a single layer, and place the lemon slices over the top.
4. Broil for 8-10 minutes.
5. Serve with the asparagus and beans/peas.

DAY 16

Breakfast: Double Chocolates Tahini Banana Muffins

Prep + Cooking time: 10 minutes

Servings: 12

Ingredients:

- 1 heaping glass mashed ripe banana (about 2-3 bananas)
- 2 large eggs
- 1/2 glass of tahini
- 1/3 cup 100% pure maple syrup
- 1 teaspoon of vanilla extract
- 3/4 cup of stuffed fine almond flour
- 1/2 glass of high quality unsweetened cocoa powder
- 1/4 glass of coconut flour
- 1 teaspoon of cooking soda
- 1/4 teaspoon of salt
- 1/2 cup of dairy products free chocolates chips

Directions:

1. Preheat oven to 350F.
2. In a sizable dish, add mashed banana, eggs, tahini, maple syrup and vanilla extract.
3. Mix until even and well put together.
4. In another medium dish, whisk almond flour, cocoa natural powder, and coconut flour, cooking soda and sodium.

5. Add dry materials to wet substances and mix materials along until well mixed. Fold in chocolates potato chips, reserving a few delicious chocolate potato chips for sprinkling together with muffins.

6. Divide batter uniformly between ready muffin liners. Bake for 18-25 minutes.

Lunch: Shrimp and Avocado Salad with Tahini Dressing

Prep + Cooking time: 15 minutes

Servings: 6

Ingredients:

- 5 mugs baby kale and baby spinach mix
- 1 medium-sized cucumber
- 1 avocado
- 1 tablespoon lime juice
- 1/2 lb. uncooked shrimp
- 3 cloves garlic clove, minced
- 1/2 teaspoon cumin
- 1/2 teaspoon Old Bay seasoning
- 1/4 teaspoon chipotle chili pepper powder
- 1/4 teaspoon cayenne pepper powder
- Cooking oil
- 3 tablespoons tahini
- 1/3 glass apple cider vinegar
- 2 tablespoons water
- 1 1/2 teaspoons minced ginger
- 2 tablespoons honey
- 2 teaspoons lime juice
- 1 clove of garlic
- Sodium and pepper to taste

Directions:

1. Heat your cooking food essential oil/fat in a skillet over medium-high temperature. Add minced garlic clove and washed shrimp. Season the shrimp in the skillet with the cumin, Old Bay, chipotle chili pepper and cayenne pepper. Wait a few seconds on each part until opaque and pinky-peach in color. Remove from warmth and reserve.

2. Separate baby kale and baby spinach mixture in the middle of your bowls. Chop the cucumber and add it to the salad. Chop the avocado and cover with 1 tablespoon of lime drink. Add these to the salad as well. Finally, chop the shrimp into bite-sized items and add it to the salad.

3. To produce the dressing, combine all materials to a blender and mix until even. Drizzle over salad as desired and help.

Dinner: Caprese Hasselback Chicken

Prep + Cooking time: 30 mins

Servings: 4

Ingredients:

- 4 large chicken breast breasts, (6 oz . each)
- 4 oz fresh mozzarella parmesan cheese, the type that will come in a log
- 2 medium Roma tomato vegetables, sliced
- 1/4 glass fresh basil, divided
- 2 tablespoon of essential olive oil
- 2 tablespoon of balsamic vinegar
- sea sodium & pepper

Directions:

1. Preheat the oven to 400F.
2. Make 5-6 deep slits in each chicken white meat, being careful never to cut altogether.
3. Cut the tomato vegetables and mozzarella very thinly, about 1/8" to 1/4" dense, and slice the items to a width somewhat more full than the width of your chicken white meat.
4. Drizzle essential olive oil and balsamic vinegar within the chicken.
5. Bake for 20-25 minutes, until appropriately cooked through.
6. Once the chicken is ready, sprinkle leftover fresh basil ribbons at the top right before serving.

DAY 17

Breakfast: Almond Flour Crepes

Prep + Cooking time: 10 minutes

Servings: 4

Ingredients:

- 4 eggs
- ¼ of glass almond meal
- 1 teaspoon of vanilla essence
- 1/4 teaspoon of surface cinnamon
- 1 tablespoon of extra virgin coconut essential oil, to grease the crepe pan

Directions:

1. Whisk the eggs, earth almond, vanilla, and cinnamon together.
2. Scoop the crepe batter into the frying skillet ,
3. Make the crepe for about 2 minutes each, over medium heating.
4. Repeat for another crepe.
5. To serve each crepe completely with the whipped coconut cream, flip in a triangle and top with the fruits of your choice.

Lunch: Easy Cashew Chicken

Prep + Cooking time: 25 minutes

Servings: 3

Ingredients:

- 3 raw fowl thighs boneless, skinless
- 2 tablespoon of canola oil
- 1/4 glass cashews
- 1/2 medium Green Bell Pepper
- 1/2 tablespoon of surface ginger
- 1 tablespoon of rice wines vinegar
- 1 1/2 tablespoon of soy sauce
- 1/2 tablespoon of chili garlic sauce
- 1 tablespoon of minced garlic
- 1 tablespoon of Sesame Olive oil
- 1 tablespoon of Sesame Seed products
- 1 tablespoon of green onions
- 1/4 medium white onion
- Sodium + Pepper

Directions:

1. Heat a skillet over low high temperature and toast the cashews for 8 minutes. Remove and reserve.
2. Dice chicken breast thighs into 1 inches chunks. Trim onion and pepper into large pieces.

3. Add essential canola oil to the pan.

4. Add the fowl thighs and leave for about 5 minutes to cook thoroughly.

5. Add the pepper, onions, garlic clove; chili garlic clove sauce and seasonings (ginger, sodium, pepper). Allow cooking for 2-3 minutes.

6. Add soy sauce, grain wines vinegar, and cashews

7. Serve in a dish, top with sesame seed products and drizzle with sesame olive oil.

Dinner: Slow Cooker Chipotle Pulled Pork

Prep + Cooking time: 8hr 10 minutes

Servings: 4

Ingredients:

- 1 Small Onion, peeled and lower into chunks
- 3 Cloves Garlic clove, peeled
- 1 Tablespoon Extra Light essential olive oil
- 1/2 Orange, juiced
- 2 Limes, juiced
- 3 Teaspoons Chipotle Pepper Powder
- 2 Teaspoons Paprika
- 1 Teaspoon Cumin
- 1 Teaspoon Oregano
- 1 Teaspoon Salt
- 1/2 Teaspoon Dark Pepper
- 1 (3-4 lb.) Pork Loin
- 1/4 Glass Chicken Broth

Directions:

1. Combine the onion, garlic clove, essential olive oil, orange drink, lime drink, and spices in a blender and pulse until mainly smooth.
2. Marinate the pork. Make sure the pork is layered well. Refrigerate the pork overnight.
3. Each day, place the pork along with marinade into the slow cooker and put in the chicken breast broth.
4. Make the pork for 8 times on low, or until you can shred it with a fork.

DAY 18

Breakfast: Cooked Denver Omelet

Prep + Cooking time: 5 minutes

Servings: 6

Ingredients:

- 1/2 cup of cut red bell pepper
- 1/2 cup of cut green bell pepper
- 1/3 cup of sliced yellow onion
- 2 tablespoon of essential olive oil
- 1 cup of cut grilled ham
- 8 large eggs
- 1/3 of glass milk
- Salt and newly ground dark pepper
- 1/2 glass of shredded sharpened cheddar cheese
- Avocados (optional)
- Chives and hot sauce(optional)

Directions:

1. Preheat oven to 400 degrees.
2. Put ham into an even layer over medium-high heating. Once hot, add red and green bell peppers and onion and cook for about 4 minutes.
3. Pour pepper concoction and sprinkle equally with cheese.
4. In a huge mixing, dish whisk eggs and dairy until well combined.
5. Season with sodium and pepper and mix.

6. Bake in preheated oven for about 22 - 25 minutes.

7. Slice and serve warm with avocado pieces and optional chives and hot sauce.

Lunch: Great Potato Spinach Soup

Prep + cooking time: 25 minutes

Servings: 6

Ingredients:

- 2 tablespoons extra-virgin essential olive oil
- 2 cloves garlic clove crushed
- 1 small onion diced
- 2 1/2 cup of potatoes peeled,
- 2 cup chopped up zucchini washed, unpeeled, about 3 minute zucchini
- 1/4 cup even Italian parsley
- 4 mugs fresh spinach leaves washed
- 4 cups veg stock
- 1 teaspoon salt
- 1 pinch chili flakes or earth pepper

Directions:

1. Warm the essential olive oil.
2. Add garlic clove and onion and prepare for 1-2 minutes.
3. Add special potatoes, zucchini, spinach leaves, parsley.
4. Make meals for 1-2 minutes.
5. Add veggie stock, cover, reduce to low heating and simmer for a quarter-hour or before vegetables are soft.
6. Pour the soup into a blender to mix.
7. Put sodium and pepper to taste.

Dinner: Sheet Skillet Roasted Asparagus & Rooster With Chorizo

Prep + cooking time: 27 minutes

Servings: 2

Ingredients:

For the onion & pepper mixture

- 1 large brownish onion, diced
- 1 medium red pepper, diced
- 1 small chorizo sausage, peeled and diced (about 100-150 g / 4-5 oz.)
- 1/2 teaspoon paprika powder
- 1/2 teaspoon onion natural powder (optional)
- 1/2 teaspoon cumin powder
- Pinch of dried out coriander or thyme
- Pinch of sodium and pepper
- 3 tablespoons essential olive oil
- 2 tablespoons lemon juice

For the chicken

- 4-5 chicken breast tenderloins, slice into 3 parts each
- 1 teaspoon paprika
- 1/4 teaspoon cumin powder
- Large pinch of salt
- 1 tablespoon essential olive oil

For asparagus

- 100 g / 3-4 oz. asparagus spears
- 2 cloves garlic clove, finely diced
- 2 tablespoons lemon juice
- 1 tablespoon essential olive oil
- Large pinch of salt

Directions:

1. Preheat oven to 410 F.
2. In the mixing bowl, your ingredients.
3. Blend the chicken elements in the same dish. Pass on the chicken bits together with the onion and peppers.
4. For the time being, incorporate the asparagus with garlic, lemon drink, essential olive oil and sodium and reserve. After ten minutes, take away the sheet skillet from the oven. Scatter the asparagus spears between the poultry and sprinkle with the rest of the garlic clove and juices. Transform the heat right down to 200 C / 400 F and place the holder back for 7 minutes. Remove from the holder and serve while hot.

DAY 19

Breakfast: Low-Carb No Egg Breakfast Baked With Sausage And Peppers

Prep + cooking time: 27 minutes

Servings: 4

Ingredients:

- 1 bell pepper
- 1 tablespoon of essential olive oil
- Spike seasoning to style
- Fresh-ground dark-colored pepper to taste
- About 10 oz. turkey or pork breakfast time sausage links
- 1/2 glass Mozzarella, grated

Directions:

1. Preheat oven to 450F/230C.
2. Put peppers into the cooking dish, toss with 1 teaspoon of essential olive oil, sprinkle with Spike Seasoning and fresh-ground dark-colored pepper, and put the dish in the oven and bake for 20 minutes.
3. Slice sausages into three.
4. Once the peppers have grilled for 20 minutes, mix in the sausages and bake five minutes more.
5. Remove from oven, turn oven to broil, sprinkle the grated Mozzarella on the sausage-pepper blend and put broil for 1-2 minutes. Serve hot.

Lunch: Keto Garlic Clove Mascarpone Broccoli Alfredo Fried Pizza

Prep + cooking time: 25 minutes

Servings: 6

Ingredients:

- 1 tablespoon of garlic essential olive oil
- 1 glass shredded pizza mozzarella cheese blend
- 1 glass shredded mozzarella cheese
- 1/4 glass mascarpone cheese
- 2 tablespoon of ghee
- 1 tablespoon of heavy cream
- 1 tablespoon of minced garlic
- 1/8 tablespoon of lemon pepper seasoning
- 2 pinches of salt
- 1/3 glass steamed, cut broccoli heads
- Shaved asiago parmesan cheese to taste

Directions:

1. Add essential olive oil and hold out until it's hot and shimmers.
2. Add pizza mozzarella cheese mix first
3. Make meals for 4-5 minutes until it gets crispy.
4. Add mascarpone parmesan cheese, ghee, heavy cream, garlic, lemon pepper and sodium to the hot skillet, and prepare until melted and commences to bubble, then remove from heating so that it doesn't break.
5. Drizzle one half the mixtures within the crust.
6. Add the cut, steamed broccoli to the spouse.

7. Cook for approximately 1 minute until hot and bubbling.

8. Add the broccoli to the pizza.

9. Sprinkle shaved asiago parmesan cheese and further lemon pepper seasoning (optional)

Dinner: Easy Cashew Chicken

Prep + cooking time: 15 minutes

Servings: 3

Ingredients:

- 3 raw chicken breast thighs boneless, skinless
- 2 tablespoon of canola oil (for baking)
- 1/4 glass cashews
- 1/2 medium Green Bell Pepper
- 1/2 teaspoon of earth ginger
- 1 tablespoon of grain wines vinegar
- 1 1/2 tablespoon of soy sauce
- 1/2 tablespoon of chili garlic sauce
- 1 tablespoon of minced garlic
- 1 tablespoon of Sesame Olive oil
- 1 tablespoon of Sesame Seed products
- 1 tablespoon of green onions
- 1/4 medium white onion
- Sodium + Pepper

Directions:

1. Heat a skillet over low high temperature and toast the cashews for 8 minutes
2. Dice chicken breast thighs into 1-inch chunks. Slice onion and pepper into even large pieces.
3. Increase temperature to high and add canola oil to the pan.
4. Add the poultry thighs for about five minutes.

5. After the chicken is thoroughly cooked. Add the pepper, onions, garlic clove, chili garlic clove sauce and seasonings (ginger, sodium, pepper). Allow cooking for 2-3 minutes.

6. Add soy sauce, grain wine beverages vinegar, and cashews.

7. Serve in a dish, top with sesame seed products and drizzle with sesame oil.

DAY 20

Breakfast: Egg Muffin Cups

Prep + cooking time: 25 minutes

Servings: 6

Ingredients:

- 2 mugs of spinach, chopped
- 1 large Roma tomato
- 1/2 glass of baby Bella mushrooms, diced
- 1 jalapeno, seeded and diced
- 12 eggs
- 1/4 glass of unsweetened almond dairy (or any dairy)
- 1/2 teaspoon salt
- Freshly ground dark pepper
- Optional: 3/4 glass of shredded cheddar cheese

Directions:

1. Preheat oven to 350F.
2. Divide spinach, tomato vegetables, mushrooms, and jalapeno to 12 muffins in the tin.
3. In a sizable bowl whisk along eggs, almond dairy, sodium, and pepper until well put together.
4. Fill up each muffin about 3/4 way full with egg mix.
5. Bake for 25-30 minutes. Remove and serve.

Lunch: Caesar Egg Salad Lettuce Wraps

Prep + cooking time: 15 minutes

Servings: 4

Ingredients:

- 6 large hard-boiled eggs, peeled and chopped
- 3 tablespoon of creamy Caesar dressing
- 3 tablespoon of mayonnaise
- 1/2 glass Parmesan parmesan cheese, shredded, divided
- Cracked dark pepper, to taste
- 4 large romaine lettuce leaves

Directions:

1. In a combining bowl, incorporate sliced eggs, creamy Caesar dressing, mayonnaise, 1/4 glass of parmesan cheese and cracked dark-colored pepper.
2. Spoon combination onto romaine leaves and top with extra Parmesan cheese.

Dinner: Bacon Wrapped Chicken Bombs

Prep + Cooking time: 45 minutes

Servings: 2

Ingredients:

- 3 boneless chicken breasts
- 15 ounces frozen spinach
- 4 ounces cream cheese, dissolved
- 1/2 cup full-fat ricotta
- Salt and pepper to taste
- Bacon 12 slices

Directions:

1. Preset the oven to 375F.
2. Mix the green spinach with the creamy mozzarella cheese and full-fat ricotta. Season with salt and pepper to taste.
3. Cut the chicken breasts in half.
4. Stuff the pouches with the cheese stuffing.
5. Wrap bacon around each piece of chicken.
6. Sear the bacon covered chicken in a hot skillet.
7. Set the bits of chicken into the safe oven dish while you prepare the rest
8. Bake for 35-45 minutes. The chicken is done when it gets to 165F.

DAY 21

Breakfast: Muesli Low Carbohydrate Cereal

Prep + Cooking time: 1 minute

Servings: 15

Ingredients:

- 1 glass of sunflower seeds
- 1 glass of unsweetened flaked coconut
- 1 glass of pumpkin seeds
- 1 cup of chopped up almonds
- 1/2 glass of pecans
- 1/2 glass of hemp hearts
- 2 teaspoons of cinnamon
- 1/2 teaspoon of vanilla extract
- 1/4 teaspoon of vanilla stevia drops

Directions:

1. In large dish, stir collectively all ingredients until well mixed.
2. Lay out over a rimmed baking skillet and bake at 350F for approximately 7-8 minutes.
3. Allow cooling.
4. Store in air small container.
5. Each serving is approximately 1/3 cup.
6. Preferences great with almond dairy!

Lunch: 5 Minute Keto Pizza

Prep + cooking time: 5 minutes

Servings: 1

Ingredients:

Pizza Crust

- 2 large Eggs
- 2 tablespoon of Parmesan Cheese
- 1 tablespoon of Psyllium Husk Powder
- 1/2 teaspoon of Italian Seasoning
- Salt to Taste
- 2 tablespoon of Frying Oil Toppings
- 1.5 oz. Mozzarella Cheese
- 3 tablespoon of Rao's Tomato Sauce
- 1 tablespoon of Newly Chopped Basil

Directions:

1. Put all dried materials into a dish or pot that can fit your immersion blender.
2. Add 2 eggs and blend everything together making use of your immersion blender. Be sure you continue mixing for approximately 30 seconds, allowing the psyllium husk to soak up a few of the liquid.
3. Heat 2 teaspoons of frying olive oil in a skillet over medium-high high temperature. Once scorching, spoon your blend into the skillet and disperse into a circle shape.
4. Once the corners have begun to set and appear slightly brown, turn the pizza crust.

5. Cook for 30-60 seconds, then put about 3 tablespoons of Rao's tomato sauce on the pizza and spread around.

6. Add parmesan cheese, then put the pizza into the oven to broil. Leave a split wide open in the oven so you will keep an eye on it. Once it's bubbling, take it off.

7. Serve with some newly chopped basil.

Dinner: Sheet Pan Pesto Chicken with Asparagus Tomatoes And Walnuts

Prep + cooking time: 35 minutes

Servings: 4

Ingredients:

- 1 1/2 mugs (48g) jam-packed fresh basil leaves
- 1/4 glass Fishers Walnuts Halves and Pieces
- 1/4 glass finely shredded parmesan cheese
- 2 cloves garlic clove , peeled
- 1/2 cup essential olive oil
- Sodium and freshly floor black pepper

Hen and Veggies

- 1 1/2 pounds boneless skinless poultry chest , diced into 1-in . pieces
- 1 lb asparagus (avoid thick spears), hard ends trimmed and discarded staying diced into 1 1/2-inches pieces
- 1 pint of fresh grape tomatoes
- 1/2 glass Fishers Walnuts Halves and Pieces

Directions:

1. Preheat oven to 400 degrees.
2. For the pesto, add basil leaves, 1/4 glass walnuts, parmesan and garlic clove to a food processor chip. Pulse until coarsely cut.
3. Add essential olive oil, season with sodium and pepper to flavor and pulse until everything is finely cut and well mixed. Set aside.

4. Brand a rimmed 18 by 13-inch baking sheet with a sheet of parchment paper or spray with non-stick cooking spray.

5. Place rooster and asparagus on sheet skillet put over 1/4 glass of the basil pesto.

6. Season chicken breast and asparagus with sodium and pepper and toss everything to coat uniformly.

7. Pass on into an even layer (don't allow chicken portions overlap) and roast in preheated oven for ten minutes.

8. Remove from oven, carefully drain off extra liquid in one place if needed.

9. Add tomato vegetables.

10. Remove from oven, spoon over another 1/4 glass of the pesto and toss. Sprinkle in walnuts.

11. Serve immediately.

DAY 22

Breakfast: Sausage Egg "Mcmuffin"

Prep + cooking time: 10 minutes

Servings: 1

Ingredients:

- 2 tablespoons of ghee
- 1/4 pound bulk raw pork breakfast time sausage
- 2 large eggs
- Kosher salt
- Freshly ground dark pepper
- 1/4 glass water
- 1 heaping tablespoon guacamole (optional)

Directions:

1. Grab two stainless 3 1/2 -inches biscuit cutters, and grease the insides well with melted ghee.
2. Place one cutter on the plate and fill it with the sausage meats.
3. Delicately press the beef right down to condition a sausage patty uniformly.
4. Heat a skillet over medium-high temperature and put in a tablespoon of ghee.
5. Once the fat is shimmering, add the patty to the skillet. In the event that you want the patty to keep its correctly round condition, you will keep the mildew on before cooked patty shrinks properly from the edges. Then, lift up it off and away.
6. Clean the biscuit cutter and grease it again.
7. Fry the sausage about 2-3 three minutes on each area or until thoroughly cooked.

8. When your patty's thick, you may want to cover the skillet to be sure it's grilled through. After the patty's ready, put it to a dish.

Lunch: Salad With Easy Italian Dressing

Prep + cooking time: 10 minutes

Servings: 3-4

Ingredients:

- 1 big head or 2 hearts romaine chopped
- 4 oz . prosciutto cut in strips
- 4 oz . salami or pepperoni cubed
- 1/2 glass of artichoke hearts sliced
- 1/2 glass of olives mixture of dark and green
- 1/2 glass of hot or cute peppers pickled or roasted

Direction:

1. Combine all materials in a huge salad dish. Toss with Italian dressing.

Dinner: Roasted Asian Shrimp And Brussels Sprouts Sheet Skillet Meal

Prep + Cooking time: 30 minutes

Servings: 4

Ingredients:

- 1 lb. jumbo iced shrimp, thawed and drained well
- 1 lb. brussels sprouts stems trimmed and minimize in half
- 1-2 T essential olive oil
- sodium and fresh-ground dark pepper to taste

Directions:

1. Thaw shrimp immediately in the refrigerator.
2. Preheat oven to 400F/200C and squirt a big cooking sheet with oil or non-stick aerosol.
3. After the shrimp have drained well, hook them up to a part of paper bath towels, cover with an increase of bath towels, and blot dried up, so these are as dry as possible get them.
4. Position the dried out shrimp and 50 percent of the marinade/glaze concoction into a Ziploc handbag.
5. Put brussels sprouts into a dish and toss with the desired amount of essential olive oil, sodium, and fresh-ground dark pepper, then roast a quarter-hour.
6. After the brussels sprouts have grilled a quarter-hour, drain the shrimp well in a colander put in the kitchen sink.
7. Roast for about 6-8 minutes until shrimp have transformed green and are scarcely strong.
8. Take away the sheet skillet from the oven, take the shrimp and brussels sprouts and serve.

DAY 23

Breakfast: Bacon And Egg Cups

Prep + Cooking time: 10 minutes

Servings: 12

Ingredients:

- 12 eggs
- 12 items nitrate free bacon (paleo approved if possible)
- 1 tablespoon of cut chives
- Sodium and pepper

Directions:

1. Preheat oven to 400 degrees.
2. Cook bacon for approximately 8-10 minutes.
3. Remove from skillet while still pliable, not crisp. Cool on paper towels.
4. Grease your muffin tins.
5. Put one little bit of bacon in each opening, wrapping it around to line the sides.
6. Split the eggs into each gap. Top with cut chives. Sodium and pepper to flavor.
7. Cook for approximately 12-15 minutes or until bacon is clean. Watch closely.

Lunch: Zucchini Crust Grilled Cheese

Prep + cooking time: 30 minutes

Servings: 2

Ingredients:

- 4 mugs of shredded zucchini
- 1 egg
- 1/2 glass shredded mozzarella cheese
- 4 tablespoons grated Parmesan cheese
- 1 teaspoon dried out oregano
- 1/2 teaspoon salt
- Pinch of earth black pepper
- Grilled cheese
- 1 tablespoon butter, room temperature
- 85 gr pointed cheddar parmesan cheese, grated/shredded, at room temperature

Directions:

1. Preheat oven to 450F.
2. Line a cooking sheet with parchment newspaper and liberally grease it. Reserve.
3. Microwave shredded zucchini for 6 minutes.
4. In a dish mix zucchini, egg, mozzarella cheese, oregano, sodium, and pepper.
5. Spread zucchini combination onto the lined cooking sheet and condition into 4 squares.
6. Bake for 15 to 20 minutes until gently golden brown.
7. Remove from the oven and let cool ten minutes before peeling them off of the parchment newspaper
8. Assemble grilled cheese

9. Heat a skillet over medium heating.

10. Butter one part of each cut of zucchini crust bread (preferably the very best part).

11. Place one cut off a loaf of bread in the skillet, buttered area down, sprinkle with the cheese and top with a zucchini crust.

12. Turn heat down a notch and make until golden brownish, about 2 to 4 minutes.

13. Gently turn and make until golden brownish on the other hand, about 2 to 4 minutes.

Dinner: Five Spice Glazed Chicken

Prep + Cooking time: 1 hr 30min

Servings: 4

Ingredients:

- 1 whole chicken
- 1/3 glass soy sauce
- 6 slices ginger
- 1 teaspoon five spice powder
- 2 tablespoons sugar-free maple syrup

Directions:

1. Mix the soy sauce, ginger pieces, and spice powder.
2. Sprinkle half of a teaspoon of the five-spice natural powder into the chicken.
3. Marinade in a single day, turning occasionally
4. Preheat your oven to 350F. Use a roasting rack to put the chicken on the baking sheet.
5. Roast with whatever fruit and vegetables you intend for 20 minutes. After that sprinkle with oil.
6. Cook for just two more 20-minute intervals, and moisten, before chicken has adequately cooked for one hour.
7. After the chicken has adequately cooked for one hour, then start moistening it every ten minutes, for another half hour. Keep checking till it reaches about 165F. Serve.

DAY 24

Breakfast: Cinnamon Spin Muffins

Prep + cooking time: 20 minutes

Servings: 2

Ingredients:

- 1/2 glass almond flour
- 2 scoops vanilla necessary protein natural powder 32-34 grams per scoop
- 1 tablespoon of cooking powder
- 1 tablespoon of cinnamon
- 1/2 glass nut or seed butter of preference almond butter, peanut butter, sunflower seed butter, etc.
- 1/2 glass pumpkin puree can sub for unsweetened applesauce, mashed banana or mashed prepared sweet potato
- 1/2 glass coconut oil

For the glaze

- 1/4 glass coconut butter
- 1/4 cup dairy of choice
- 1 tablespoon of granulated sweetener of preference
- 2 tablespoon of lemon juice

Directions:

1. Preheat in the oven to 350F
2. In a sizable mixing bowl, ingredients and combination well.

3. Bake the muffins for 10-15 minutes,

4. Allow cooling in skillet for five minutes, before moving to a cable rack to cool completely.

5. Once cooled, ready your cinnamon and mix it with other ingredients.

6. Drizzle in the muffin tops and serve.

Lunch: Keto Rooster Enchilada Bowl

Prep + cooking time: 30 minutes

Servings: 4-6

Ingredients:

- 2-3 chicken chest
- 3/4 mugs red enchilada sauce
- 1/4 glass water
- 1/4 glass onion
- 1 4 oz can green chilies
- 1 12oz steam tote cauliflower rice
- Roma tomatoes
- Seasoning, to taste

Directions:

1. Cook chicken chest until casually brown
2. Add enchilada sauce, chilies, onions, drinking water and reduce temperature to simmer
3. Cover and prepare food until chicken is grilled through
4. Add chicken back to the sauce and continue simmering for ten more minutes uncovered or until almost all of the water has been assimilated
5. Prepare cauliflower grain and dice preferred toppings
6. Top grain with chicken, parmesan cheese, avocado or preferred toppings

Dinner: Keto Stuffed Meatloaf

Prep + Cooking time: 1 hr

Servings: 6

Ingredients:

- 500 grams of well-grounded beef
- 6 pieces cheddar cheese
- 1/4 cup sliced onions
- 1/4 cup cut green onions
- 1/2 glass spinach
- 1/4 glass mushrooms

Directions:

1. Mix the well-grounded beef with the sodium, pepper, garlic clove, and cumin.
2. Layer the mozzarella cheese underneath of the meatloaf.
3. Add the onions, spinach, and mushrooms.
4. Utilize the leftover meat to put on top, with the spinach and mushrooms, operating as a cover.
5. Bake at 350F for just one hour.

DAY 25

Breakfast: French Toast - Almond Turmeric Cricket Bread

Prep + cooking time: 10 minutes

Servings: 4

Ingredients:

- 8 pieces Gluten-Free Paleo Cricket Tumeric Bread
- 2 eggs
- 3/4 glass coconut milk
- 1/2 teaspoon floor cinnamon
- 2 tablespoons coconut sugar
- 1 tablespoon vanilla essence
- 1 teaspoon extra virgin coconut oil

Toppings

- 1 banana sliced
- 6 fresh strawberries
- 3 tablespoon maple syrup or honey

Directions:

1. Whisk together eggs, coconut dairy, surface cinnamon, coconut glucose, vanilla essence.
2. Heat a skillet or crepe skillet under medium temperature.
3. Add 1/2 teaspoon of coconut for 4 bakery slices.

4. Dunk each cut of paleo bread in the egg mix, soaking both sides. Put it in the hot skillet, and make on both sides until golden. With regards to the bread you are using, you might have to add a little bit more coconut olive oil.

5. Add 1/2 teaspoon at the same time and observe how it goes.

6. Serve hot with banana pieces, fresh strawberries and a drizzle of maple syrup or honey.

Lunch: Guacamole Rooster Salad

Prep + cooking time: 10 minutes

Servings: 2-3

Ingredients:

- 2 large avocados
- 1 tablespoon of freshly-squeezed lime juice
- 1 glass cilantro, chopped
- 1/4-1/2 glass red onion, finely chopped
- 2-3 ribs celery, finely cut (about 1/2 glass)
- 2 large serrano chili peppers, finely chopped
- 1 teaspoon kosher salt
- 2 cooked chicken chest, epidermis removed
- Butter lettuce leaves, for serving

Directions:

1. Mash avocados with a citrus drink in a tiny dish. Add cilantro, cut onion, serrano chili peppers, and sodium. Stir to mix.
2. Serve with lettuce leaves.

Dinner: Sausage Zucchini Boats

Prep + Cooking time: 1 hour

Servings: 2

Ingredients:

- 2 medium zucchini
- 1 pound earth sausage
- 1 glass shredded cheddar cheese
- 1/2 medium onion, chopped
- 1 tablespoon minced garlic
- 1 teaspoon paprika
- 1/2 teaspoon red pepper flakes
- 1 teaspoon dried out oregano
- 1/2 cup chicken breast broth
- Sodium and pepper to taste

Directions:

1. Trim your zucchini in two.
2. Scoop out the zucchini so that it becomes a shell for the fillings.
3. Chop up the zucchini that you scooped from the skins.
4. In a skillet saute your onions, garlic clove, and scooped zucchini on medium heating.
5. Turn heat up to medium-high then add the sausage.
6. After the sausage has adequately cooked, blend in your parmesan cheese, until it melts.
7. Divide the cooked zucchini and sausage equally among the zucchini shells.
8. Top with parmesan cheese and place into a casserole dish.
9. Pour 1/2 glass of chicken broth into the dish.

10. Bake at 350F for thirty minutes.

DAY 26

Breakfast: Easy Spinach & Mushroom Omelet Muffins

Prep + Cooking time: 5 minutes

Servings: 15

Ingredients:

- 1/4 glass of butter
- 8 oz. mushrooms sliced
- Sodium and pepper
- 2 cloves garlic clove minced
- 5 oz . fresh spinach
- 2/3 glass of Bob's Red Mill coconut flour
- 2 tablespoon of cooking powder
- 3/4 tablespoon of salt
- 1/2 tablespoon of pepper
- 7 large eggs
- 1/2 glass of whipping cream
- 1 cup of grated cheese of choice

Directions:

1. Set oven to 350F. This menu makes about 15 muffins so you might need to work in batches if you merely have one muffin skillet.
2. In a sizable saute skillet, melt butter over medium heating.
3. Once hot and melted, add sliced up mushrooms.
4. After 1 minute add sodium and pepper to tastes and sauté until gold darkish.

5. Add garlic clove for 30 secs, then add the new spinach. Make until just wilted, about 1 more minute. Reserve.

6. In a huge bowl, whisk the coconut flour, cooking powder, sodium, and pepper collectively. Add eggs, whipping cream and grated parmesan cheese and whisk until well blended. Mix in mushroom/spinach concoction.

7. Spoon batter into well-prepared muffin mugs to about 3/4 full. Bake for 25 to 30 minutes.

Lunch: Spinach Cobb Salad Recipe

Prep + Cooking time: 10 minutes

Servings: 2

Ingredients:

- 2 cups fresh baby spinach
- 4 oz. prepared chicken
- 1/3 cup sliced cucumber
- 1/3 cup cut tomatoes
- 2 large hard-boiled eggs
- 1/4 lb. good quality bacon, grilled and crumbled
- 1/2 large avocado, minimize into small chunks

Directions:

1. Place your spinach in a dish.
2. Top with all of those other elements and add the dressing of your decision.

Dinner: Jalapeño Popper Pizza

Prep + Cooking time: 40 minutes

Servings: 2

Ingredients:

Crust

- 2 cups disposed of mozzarella cheese
- 3/4 mugs almond flour
- 1/2 tablespoon oregano
- 1/2 teaspoon paprika
- 1/2 teaspoon red soup flakes

Toppings

- 1 teaspoon tomato paste
- ¾ cup sausage pieces
- ½ cup chopped jalapeno potatoes
- 11 teaspoon cream dairy products
- 1/2 teaspoon garlic herb powdered
- 3 tablespoons cut chives

Directions:

1. In a microwave-safe bowl, place your mozzarella cheese. Add other ingredients.
2. Heat the cheese up in the microwave, for approximately one minute.
3. Stir your almond flour into the cheese.
4. Place your dough on a pizza tray, knead the bread together.

5. Roll the edges of the dough towards the center of the pizza to make a crust.

6. Place a scrap of tomato paste on the dough, spreading it around.

7. Using a teaspoon, place 1/2 chunks of cream cheese around the pizzas. Top with jalapenos, bread, chives, and natural garlic powder.

8. Cook at 350F for 30-40 minutes.

DAY 27

Breakfast: Savory Chicken Sausage

Prep + Cooking time: 20 minutes

Servings: 12

Ingredients:

- 8 large eggs
- 1/2 glass unsweetened almond milk
- 1/2 teaspoon salt
- Freshly ground dark pepper
- 1/3 glass coconut flour
- 1/2 pound of chicken sausage of preference
- 1 glass of shredded cheddar mozzarella cheese, divided (use whatever cheese you prefer)

Directions:

1. Preheat oven to 400F. Generously grease 12 muffin mugs of a muffin tin with nonstick food preparation spray.
2. In the medium dish, whisk the eggs, almond dairy, sodium, and pepper. Gradually add coconut flour, while still whisking.
3. Collapse in cooked hen sausage and 1/2 glass of shredded cheese.
4. Evenly pour combination into the greased muffin tins.
5. Sprinkle with 1/2 glass of remaining mozzarella cheese.
6. Bake for a quarter-hour.

Lunch: Eggplant Pizza Bites - Low Carbohydrate + Keto

Prep + Cooking time: 25 minutes

Servings: 10

Ingredients:

- 1 eggplant, trimmed, minimize in thick pieces, skin on
- 1/2 teaspoon coarse sea salt

Toppings

- 3/4 glass tomato pasta
- 1/2 glass grated mozzarella cheese
- 1/3 glass baby spinach leaves
- 10 cherry tomatoes
- 1 teaspoon garlic essential olive oil - optional
- 1 teaspoon dried out oregano

Directions:

1. Preheat your oven to 220C (425 F)
2. Prepare a cooking sheet protected with parchment newspaper and set up the eggplant pieces on the sheet. Make sure they don't really overlap or touch one another.
3. Sprinkle the coarse sea sodium on top. Reserve for ten minutes. Then bake for a quarter-hour at 220C (425F).
4. Remove the cooked eggplant pieces from the oven, flip within the eggplant pieces and swap the oven to broil/barbeque grill mode.
5. Brush some garlic clove olive oil together with each eggplant pieces
6. Spread in regards to a tablespoon of tomato sauce over each eggplant pieces.

7. Then, add your chosen toppings: few baby spinach leaves, grated mozzarella cheese, and 50 percent cherry tomatoes.

8. Put in a sprinkle of dried out the oregano and go back to the oven, broil function, for 3-5 minutes or before parmesan cheese is grilled and melted.

9. Serve immediately.

Dinner: Rich And Creamy Beef Casserole

Prep + Cooking time: 25 minutes

Servings: 3

Ingredients:

- 16 ounces cauliflower grain
- 5 pounds 80/20 ground beef
- 15 oz . green enchilada spices
- 0.5 cup sour cream
- 0.25 cups small curd bungalow cheese
- 2 cups destroyed cheddar cheese
- 1/2 glass sliced green onions
- Salt
- 1 teaspoons black pepper

Directions:

1. Preheat oven to 350F. Place the cauliflower rice into a microwave bowl then cook for 4-5 minutes until it softened.
2. Brown the meat over medium-high heat. Serve in the green enchilada sauce, then season with salt.
3. Add the sour cream, cottage cheese and green onions to the bowl with the cauliflower. Mix together well.
4. Place the cauliflower mixture into a casserole dish and spread out into an even layer.
5. Top the cauliflower with half of the beef mixture.
6. Create another layer with the rest of the beef, and another layer of the staying cheddar cheese.

7. Bake for 20 minutes at 450F.

DAY 28

Breakfast: Keto Breakfast Sandwich

Prep + Cooking time: 5 minutes

Servings: 1

Ingredients:

- 2 sausage patties
- 1 egg
- 1 tablespoon of cream cheese
- 2 tablespoon of distinct cheddar
- 1/4 medium avocado, sliced
- 1/4-1/2 tablespoon of sriracha (to style)
- Sodium, pepper to taste

Directions:

1. In a skillet over medium-high temperature, make sausages according to instructions and set aside.
2. In normal size bowl place cream cheese and sharp cheddar.
3. Microwave for 20-30 seconds until melted.
4. Mix mozzarella cheese with sriracha, reserve.
5. Combine egg with seasoning and make a small omelet.
6. Fill up an omelet with cheese sriracha mix and assemble the sandwich.

Lunch: Keto Tortang Talong

Prep + Cooking time: 5 minutes

Servings: 4

Ingredients:

- 4 tablespoons coconut oil
- 3 pieces Chinese eggplant
- 500 g floor beef
- 3 large eggs
- 1 fresh onions
- 1 clove garlic
- 1 small plum tomato
- 1 teaspoon dried out oregano
- 1 teaspoon floor cumin
- 1 teaspoon surface coriander
- 1 teaspoon earth paprika
- 2 teaspoons salt
- 1/3 cup sliced cilantro
- 3 teaspoons smashed pork rinds

Direction:

1. Broil eggplant and reserve.
2. In a dish beat the egg then reserve.
3. Melt 1 tablespoon coconut oil in a non-stay skillet over medium-high temperature. Saute scallions, garlic clove, and tomato until aromatic.
4. Add oregano, cumin, coriander, paprika, and sodium.

5. Add ground meat. Cook until nearly but barely grilled

6. Make an opening in the center of the eggplant.

7. Utilizing a fork, flatten and broaden the sides.

Dinner: Salted Egg Yolk And Curry Leaf Range Baked Chicken Breast Lollipop

Prep + Cooking time: 50 minutes

Servings: 2

Ingredients:

- 780 grams skin-on rooster drumettes
- 1 teaspoon kosher salt
- 1/2 teaspoon fresh surface black pepper
- 1 teaspoons cooking powder
- 3 tablespoons salted butter
- 1 tablespoon coconut oil
- 2 cloves garlic clove, crushed
- 10 medium curry leaves
- 2 tablespoons salted duck egg yolk powder
- 1 medium red bird's eyesight chili

Directions:

1. Sort out the eggs. Reserve the whites for another use.
2. Sprinkle salt on the yolk and refrigerate instantly.
3. When prepared to use, rinse out the salt with cold operating water
4. Bake yolk for ten minutes at 300F. Remove, mash, and take back to the oven to prepare food for another five minutes.
5. Transfer prepared egg yolks to a food processor chip and pulse until fine.
6. Put into the oven to dry and become powder form.
7. Store within an airtight box and refrigerate if not used immediately.

Chicken Lollipops

1. Using sharpened kitchen shears, clip the skin from the drumettes.

2. Gently season with sodium and pepper. Cover in baking natural powder.

3. Lay over a greased rack. Refrigerate for at the least 4 hours, best overnight. Once the lollipops feel "tacky," they're ready for cooking.

4. Bake at 450F for 30-35 minutes. Once done, flip, and bake for another 10-15 minutes.

Salted Egg Yolk and Curry Sauce

1. Over medium heating, melt butter, and coconut essential oil. Add garlic clove and sliced up chili. Make until aromatic. Add salted egg yolk natural powder.

2. Add curry leaves.

3. Serve altogether. Enjoy!

DAY 29

Breakfast: 4-Ingredient Flourless Low Carb Waffles

Prep + Cooking time: 5 minutes

Servings: 4

Ingredients:

- 4 large Egg
- 1/2 glass Almond butter
- 1 tablespoon of Erythritol (or any sweetener of preference)
- 1/2 tablespoon of Gluten-free cooking powder

Directions:

1. Blend all elements in a blender or food processor chip, or in a dish utilizing a palm mixer, until even.
2. Preheat in line with the manufacturer instructions. And pour about half the mixture consistently into the mixing machine and close.
3. Follow maker instructions to complete baking.
4. Repeat step 2 with the remaining batter.

Lunch: Salmon Lettuce Mugs With Lemony Basil Spread

Prep + Cooking time: 2 mins

Servings: 1

Ingredients:

- 2 leaves Boston lettuce, washed
- 1 teaspoon lemon juice
- 1/4 ounce (~6 leaves) fresh basil, finely chopped
- 1/2 teaspoon garlic clove powder
- 4 tablespoons mayonnaise
- 5-ounce of green salmon, drained
- 1/2 medium avocado, cubed
- 1 ounce chopped up red onion
- 2 tablespoons shaved Parmesan cheese

Directions:

1. Clean and ready your lettuce mugs
2. Add the lemon drink, finely sliced basil, and garlic clove powder. Mix to layer the basil leaves with the seasoning evenly.
3. Add mayonnaise and combine well. Reserve to allow flavor mix together!
4. Load the lettuce mugs with 1/2 glass of salmon each, accompanied by the cubed avocado and onion pieces.
5. Distribute the basil mayo (about 2 tbsp per portion) on the salmon and top with Parmesan cheese.

Dinner: Spaghetti Squash Lasagna Casserole

Prep + Cooking time: 60 minutes

Servings: 3

Ingredients:

- 1 whole spaghetti squash
- 2 tablespoons essential olive oil, divided
- Onions
- ground beef
- 1 tablespoon minced garlic herb
- 24 ounces Rao's marinara sauce
- 20 ounces complete milk ricotta
- 2 large eggs
- 3/4 cup roughly grated Parmesan cheese, divided
- 2 tablespoons chopped tulsi
- 0.5 teaspoon salt
- 1/2 teaspoons pepper
- 8 ounces sliced up mozzarella cheese
- 2 tablespoons chopped parsley

Directions:

1. Preheat the oven to 400F.
2. Carefully divided the spaghetti squash. Sprinkle with oil, salt, and pepper.
3. Beef roasts for 35-45 minutes
4. While the squash roasts, heat the remaining tablespoon of essential olive oil in a large skillet. Add the chopped onion, chicken, ground beef and garlic clove.

137

5. Cook the meat completely.

6. Add the marinara sauce to the various meats mixture and bring to a boil. Reduce the heat and simmer the sauce for approximately 12-15 minutes.

7. As the meat simmers incorporate the ricotta cheese, 1/2 glass Parmesan cheese, eggs, tulsi and 1/2 teaspoon sodium and pepper in a medium-sized bowl and set aside.

8. Turn the oven right down to 350F and lightly grease a 2. 5-quart casserole dish.

9. Start with spaghetti, adding half the shreds (about 2 cups) to the bottom of the dish and pressing into a flat layer.

10. Increase half the ricotta combination, followed by half the meat sauce, and a layer of half the mozzarella cheese.

11. Repeat the layers again, starting over with another layer of squash.

12. Sprinkle the casserole with the rest of the 1/4 glass of Parmesan cheese and chopped parsley.

13. Bake for 30 minutes. Take away the foil and bake another 20 - 30 minutes or until bubbly and gold brown. Serve after 15 minutes.

DAY 30

Breakfast: Coconut Flour Porridge Breakfast Time Cereal Menu

Prep + Cooking time: 2 mins

Servings: 1

Ingredients:

- 2 tablespoons coconut flour
- 2 tablespoons gold flax meal
- 3/4 glass water
- pinch of salt
- 1 large egg, beaten
- 2 teaspoons butter or ghee
- 1 tablespoon heavy cream or coconut milk
- 1 tablespoon Sukrin Yellow metal or your chosen sweetener

Directions:

1. Gauge the first four substances into a tiny container over medium heating and mix.
2. Take away the coconut flour porridge from heat and add the beaten egg, a one half at the same time, while whisking regularly.
3. Place back again on heat and continue steadily to whisk before porridge thickens.
4. Remove from heat and continue steadily to whisk for approximately 30 minutes before adding the butter, cream, and sweetener.
5. Garnish with your chosen toppings.

Lunch: Tomato Asiago Soup

Prep + Cooking time: 10 minutes

Servings: 1

Ingredients:

- 1 can of tomato paste
- 1 glass of cream
- 3/4 glass shredded Asiago cheese
- 1/4 glass water
- 1 teaspoon oregano
- 1 teaspoon minced garlic
- Sodium and pepper to taste

Directions:

1. Place your tomato paste, minced onion, and garlic clove into a container.
2. Turn on heat to medium and put in your cream.
3. Bring to a boil when you whisk the combination together.
4. Once it's boiling, add your Asiago mozzarella cheese over time. It will start thickening up. Add this and prepare food for yet another 4-5 minutes.
5. Top with pepper. Then add green onions too.

Dinner: Fast Pot White Chicken Soups

Prep + Cooking time: 30 minutes

Servings: 2

Ingredients:

- 2 tablespoons butter
- 1 medium red onion, diced
- 10 medium boneless skinless chicken thighs, cubed
- 14 ounces canned diced green chilies
- 2 teaspoons salt
- 2 teaspoons cumin
- 2 teaspoons oregano
- black pepper
- frozen cauliflower
- 4 cups chicken broth
- 2 cups sour cream
- 1 cup of heavy turning cream

Directions:

1. Melt the spread.
2. Add the diced red onion and cubed chicken.
3. Make until the chicken appears mostly done.
4. Add the green chilies, salt, cumin, oregano, black pepper, and frozen cauliflower. Stir jointly.
5. Add the 4 glasses of chicken broth. Close up the instant pot then cook on high-pressure for 30 minutes.

6. Leave for 10 minutes.

7. Whisk in the cream. Serve immediately.

88115324R00082

Made in the USA
San Bernardino, CA
10 September 2018